Effective Swiss Ball Training

Dr Paul Hermann - Osteopath
Volume 1: Functional Swiss Ball Training

Publishers Notes

For information contact,

Stay Tuned Sports Medicine
Tormore Road, Boronia
VIC, Australia 3155.
+61 03 9762 3133
www.staytuned.com.au

Printed in Australia, November 2001.

The author has made every effort to assure that the
information in this book is accurate and current at the time
of printing. The publisher and author take no responsibility
for the use of the material in this book and can not be held
responsible for any typographical or other errors found.

Please always consult your physician before initiating this
or any other exercise program. The information in this
book is not intended to replace medical advice.

Book design by: Photographs by:
The Creative Factor.   Quinn Rooney Photography
Jacob Mitchell   Melbourne, Australia
Melbourne, Australia

Danni:

My inspiration, my motivation and my best friend.
Thankyou for being such a special part of my life.

Ordering Information

For information contact:

Stay Tuned Sports Medicine
Tormore Road, Boronia
VIC, Australia 3155.
Ph: +61 03 9762 3133
Fax: +61 03 9720 6168
Web: www.staytuned.com.au

Acknowledgments

Family and friends:

Thankyou for your support and encouragement, during the writing of this book.

Index

Index

Effective Swiss Ball Training

Swiss Ball Exercises

Index

Effective Swiss Ball Training

Index

Effective Swiss Ball Training

Index

Index

Effective Swiss Ball Training

About the Author

Paul is one of Australia's leading specialists in Swiss Ball Training and Exercise Rehabilitation. He is a practising Osteopath and the owner/director of Stay Tuned Sports Medicine. He has been in the Health and Fitness industry for over 12 years working as a Gym Instructor, Personal Trainer and Coordinator of an exercise rehabilitation program.

His passion for Swiss Balls was ignited whilst completing his Masters in Osteopathy studying the Effectiveness of Swiss Ball Training on Lower Back Stability. He has since been a regular presenter in Australia and abroad at various conferences, and regularly conducts workshops and courses both nationally and internationally. Paul has also written several articles for fitness magazines and is currently involved in more research into the potential benefits of Swiss Balls.

Paul still works as a Personal Trainer and Osteopath with many elite level athletes amongst his patients at his clinic in Melbourne and regularly travels abroad to look after a variety of elite athletes and sporting groups.

Paul has been an exercise adviser to the International Diabetes Institute in Melbourne, Australia and is a lecturer in Exercise Rehabilitation, in the Osteopathic Medicine Department of RMIT University, Melbourne, Australia.

Swiss Ball training can help improve your strength, fitness, flexibility, balance, coordination and muscle tone! Just sitting on a Swiss Ball will strengthen postural muscles and improve your balance. By using your Swiss Ball for exercise you can effectively improve the strength, tone and flexibility of nearly every muscle in your body.

Swiss Balls were invented in 1909 in Switzerland by Dr. Susanne Klien-Vogelback. Dr Vogelback found that when her patients sat on a Swiss Ball they mentioned the next day that their postural muscles felt sore and tired. From this discovery Dr.Vogelback postulated that sitting on a Swiss Ball may strengthen and improve postural muscles and therefore possibly help correct postural deficiencies.

Swiss Balls are used today by many elite level athletes and teams for injury prevention and rehabilitation. Many athletes and sports teams now use Swiss Ball programs to improve their strength, tone flexibility, and motor control.

Swiss Balls themselves have not really changed much since the 1900's except the balls of today are made of strong, lightweight materials. There are several brands and types of Swiss Balls on the market today. The quality and price of these balls vary a great deal. When looking for your Swiss Ball there are a few things to keep in mind. Some balls are tested to be 'anti burst' to different pressures. This means that if you are sitting on your ball and it happens to be attacked by a pin it shouldn't burst and leave you flat on your buttocks, but will slowly deflate giving you time to get off safely. This may be very important if you rehabilitating from an injury or have a spinal condition.

Another factor to consider is the thickness and quality of the materials used in the ball. Some lower priced balls are made of thinner material that may stretch after a period of time, leaving you effectively sitting on a soft bean bag. This may result in you having to put more air in your ball to keep it firm, leaving you with a ball that is too big. The higher quality balls are made of good quality, strong materials that will maintain the ball's shape and firmness for a long time.

The way a Swiss Ball works is by teaching your body to correct itself on an unbalanced ball. That is, it trains your muscles and joints to make small corrections to movements that may put you off balance. This is what we term 'Dynamic Stability' which is the ability to maintain good postural alignment and a stable spine while it is in motion. By using minor muscular contractions and small joint adjustments the Swiss Ball will train you to stay balanced and in control of your body.

Our spines were not designed to be static and don't appreciate being still all day. This is unfortunately the case in many office workers lives. This is why many people today are replacing their chairs with Swiss Balls to keep their spines moving all day. If you choose to do this be sure to check with your Occupational Health and Safety Officer first.

Swiss Ball training helps to improve what is termed, 'Core control'. The core incorporates the section of your body between your lower ribs and the top of your pelvis and goes from your belly button through to your back. It includes all the muscles, bones, ligaments and tendons within this area.

The concept of core control is associated with "Trunk Stabilisation' and is related to the stability of your lumbar spine. Improving core control has been a goal of many rehabilitation programs for back injuries.

In basic terms core control is the ability the body has to control the muscles around your abdomen and spine and the ability this gives the body to control upper and lower limb movements. The core initiates, controls, and finishes all functional movements of your upper and lower limbs. By improving your 'Core Control' you can effectively improve the functional and athletic movements of your upper and lower limbs.

Functional Swiss Ball Training

Functional training is a method of training which uses the person's body, or parts of their body, as resistance to muscular contractions or movements. This is compared to traditional resistance training that uses weights, cables or bands as the resistance. An example of a functional exercise for the biceps muscles is a chin up as opposed to a traditional weight resisted biceps curl. The benefits of functional training is that you can train a body segment to strengthen a particular movement rather than just purely strengthen a muscle.

In general, functional training involves very little equipment and attempts to use your muscles and joints in a similar way to which they are used in everyday life. Functional training is involved in the latter stage of all rehabilitation programs and has been used to improve people's ability to perform daily functional activities with increased ease and efficiency.

High level athletes have found improvements in performance by using functional training to enable them to perform complex dynamic movements. The best example of this is a gymnast on the Roman Rings apparatus. Nearly every element of a routine on this apparatus is a complex functional movement. All the exercises in this book have been designed to be as functional as possible and none of the exercises require any equipment apart from a Swiss Ball.

By performing the functional Swiss Ball exercises in this book you will discover increases in the strength and control of the muscles in your core and your entire body. This will help you perform your daily activities with increased ease and efficiency. If you are an athlete this type of training will improve your core control giving you a stronger and more stable base for your upper and lower limb activities to work from. The improvements in your athletic skill performance may astound you.

Swiss Ball training has developed a great deal over the last 90 or so years. I am constantly inventing and trying new exercises. It is not uncommon for my friends and clients to see me flat on my nose after trying these new exercises. Most of my ideas for new exercises come from children.

Children have great functional ability because of their size and relative strength. A child playing with a Swiss Ball will unknowingly invent some of the most interesting and fun exercises which are sometimes very challenging to us mere adults. There are currently hundreds of exercises that can be performed with the Swiss Ball and this number continues to grow. Our imagination (and possibly the strength of my nose) will be the only limitation to the final number of exercises invented.

Please Note: Those people who are suffering any injury or medical condition which may compromise their ability to balance should seek guidance from their health practitioner as to whether Swiss Ball training is suitable.

Which size ball is right for you?

This is a common question which is not simple to answer. Getting the right size ball is not as simple as determining your height and picking a ball off the shelf. It is difficult to therefore match a person's height with the appropriate ball height. If you take 5 people all who are 167cm tall they may not all use the same size ball depending on their leg length and weight. A heavier person will cause the ball to displace more and may need a bigger or firmer ball.

There are a few general guides to follow when sizing a ball to use as both a chair and for exercising. When you sit on the ball with your knees directly over your heels, your hip bones should be at the same height or slightly higher than your knees. That is, your thighs should be parallel with the floor or angled slightly down towards your knees.

Another thing to remember when sizing your ball is to make sure when it is at the correct height that it is firm to sit on and does not displace too much. A softer ball will not force you to react as much and will leave you effectively sitting on a bean bag. This is why it is sometimes more suitable to purchase a slightly smaller ball and inflate it fully to ensure it is firm and still at the correct height.

As you can see very person really should be individually sized for their ball but the following guide may give you a starting point:

45cm Ball -		up to 5'	(152cm) tall
55cm Ball -	5'	up to 5'8"	(152 - 172cm) tall
65cm Ball -	5'6"	up to 6'2"	(167 - 188cm) tall
75cm Ball -	6'	up to 6'8"	(183 - 203cm) tall

Exercise Guidelines

Effective Swiss Ball Training

It is very important that before commencing this or any other exercise program, that you consult your health practitioner. The exercises in this book have been designed to increase in difficulty as you progress through the book. This is only a guide and some people may find certain exercises easier than others. Some exercises have notes on how to progress that particular exercise so if you are focusing on a particular part of the body you can use these notes to progress that exercise. If you are unsure of which exercises are suitable for you, please contact your local fitness or health professional.

All exercises in this book have been designed with safety in mind and all care has been taken in the instruction of each exercise. Due to the nature of Swiss Ball training however, some exercises may not be suitable for certain people and therefore no responsibility can be taken if injuries occur whilst you are training. Always be careful and if you are unsure or experience any discomfort when attempting an exercise please stop and consult your health practitioner before continuing.

One reason Swiss Ball training is so effective is that it causes you to exercise in an unstable environment. This forces you to react and move on the ball to maintain your balance. When exercising or even sitting on the Swiss Ball, reactive movements should be encouraged. You should feel what the ball is doing and react to it.

Continually adjusting on the ball will make you contract and strengthen muscles, improve joint mobility and increase your circulation.

Exercise Guidelines

Once an exercise becomes easy you can make it more challenging by making it harder to stay balanced on the ball. This can be achieved by bringing your feet or hands which are on the ground closer together, lifting one supporting limb off the ball or ground or just closing your eyes.

This can be demonstrated by feeling the difference in difficulty between sitting on the Swiss Ball with your feet shoulder width apart, and sitting on the ball with one leg in the air and your eyes closed.

By using this rule it is easy to progress any exercise on the Swiss Ball. Following this rule means that you will always be able to easily progress any exercise to make it more challenging and therefore obtain greater and more consistent results.

Swiss Ball Exercises

Sitting on Ball

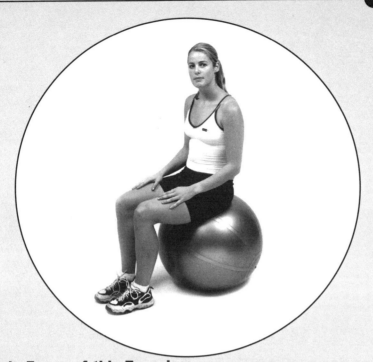

Main Focus of this Exercise:
• Core control.
• Balance.

How to perform this Exercise:
• Simply sit on the ball.
• React to the ball's movements with your pelvis to focus on core stability and spinal muscular control.
• React to the ball's movements with your ankles to focus on ankle balance and proprioception.

Notes:
• Be dynamic and react to the ball's movements.
• Keep your arms by your side or across your lap to reduce your arm movements and encourage pelvic reactions.
• Remember to look straight ahead.

Progressions:
• As you improve, move your feet closer together.
• When you can perform this exercise with control and correct postural alignment try closing your eyes or proceed to Seated One Leg Lifts.

Ab Tucks

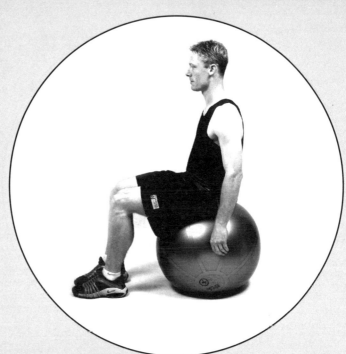

Main Focus of this Exercise:
• Increasing flexion and extension through your lumbar spine.
• Abdominal muscle control.

How to perform this Exercise:
• Start by sitting on the ball.
• Slowly tilt your pelvis back as if you are trying to stick your buttocks out.
• Bring your pelvis back to a neutral position and then slowly tilt it forward allowing your lumbar spine to flex.
• Repeat this slowly keeping the rest of your spine in a neutral postural alignment.

Notes:
• The most important thing to remember with this exercise is control.
• Keep the movements slow.
• If you are recovering from a back injury or have a chronic back condition remember to keep your movements within a pain free range of motion.

Progressions:
• When you are satisfied with the range of motion achieved and the control you have through that range, attempt the Seated Circles exercise or attempt to combine this exercise with the Seated One Leg Lifts or Seated Straight Leg Lifts exercises.

Seated Side Shifts - Level 1

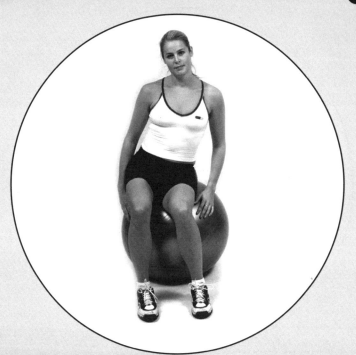

Main Focus of this Exercise:
- Core control.
- Lumbar Spine mobility.
- Pelvic and Hip mobility.

How to perform this Exercise:
- Sit on ball with feet shoulder width apart.
- Shift your pelvis to the left and right slowly as far as you can comfortably.

Notes:
- Move slowly with good control.
- Keep your spine neutral between flexion and extension.
- Keep your shoulders level.

Progressions:
- As you improve bring your feet closer together or try lifting one leg whilst moving.

Swiss Ball Exercises

Effective Swiss Ball Training

Seated Circles

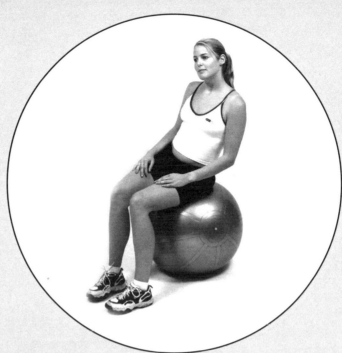

Main Focus of this Exercise:
• Spinal mobility.
• Core control.
• Dynamic balance.

How to perform this Exercise:
• Start by sitting on the ball.
• At first, think of this exercise as four separate movements.
• Firstly, push your hips out to the side, then to the back, then to the other side and finally let your pelvis tilt and push your hips to the front.
• Once you feel comfortable, put these movements together in a slow controlled circular movement.
• Keep your shoulders level and rotate from your waist only.
• Change directions each set.

Notes:
• This is sometimes called the belly dancer exercise.
• Try to keep your head still and only rotate from your waist like a belly dancer.
• React to the ball's movements as you move.
• Keep your arms across your lap or chest to reduce your arm movements and encourage pelvic reactions.

Progressions:
• As you improve, move your pelvis through larger circles or bring your feet closer together to create a narrower base of support.
• Once you can perform this exercise with good control and a good range of movement try to perform it whilst lifting one leg off the ground.
• When this becomes easy attempt it combined with a Seated Straight Leg Lift exercise or with your eyes closed.

Seated One Leg Lifts

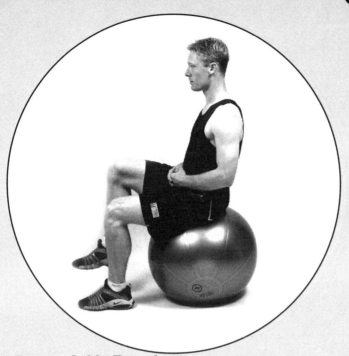

Main Focus of this Exercise:
• Core control.
• Balance.

How to perform this Exercise:
• Sit on the ball.
• Lift one leg off the ground.
• Return your leg to the ground and repeat with your other leg.

Notes:
• Be dynamic and react to the ball's movements.
• Keep your arms by your side or across your lap to reduce your arm movements and encourage pelvic reactions.
• Remember to look straight ahead.
• Keep your pelvis level.

Progressions:
• When you can perform this exercise with good control whilst maintaining correct postural alignment attempt to perform it with your eyes closed or progress to Seated Straight Leg Lifts.

Seated March

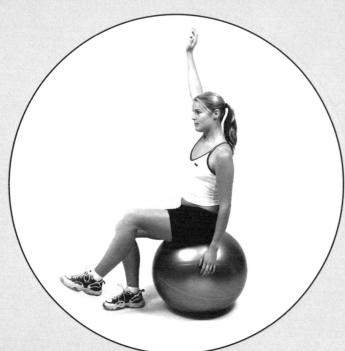

Main Focus of this Exercise:
• Core control.
• Balance.

How to perform this Exercise:
• Sit on the ball and lift your alternate arm and leg in a marching fashion slowly.

Notes:
• Be dynamic and react to the ball's movements.
• Remember to look straight ahead.

Progressions:
• As your balance and coordination improve, slow down the march to increase the time spent on each leg.
• To make this more challenging try closing your eyes whilst marching.

Seated Straight Leg Lifts - Level 1

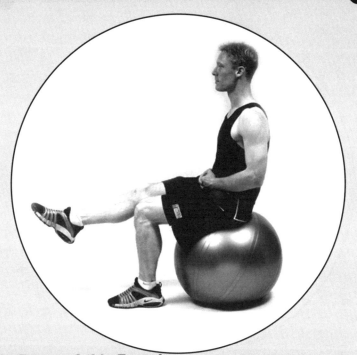

Main Focus of this Exercise:
• Core control.
• Dynamic balance.

How to perform this Exercise:
• Sit on the ball.
• Lift one leg off ground.
• Straighten out your leg.
• Hold your leg in the air whilst maintaining your balance on the ball.
• Return your leg to the ground and repeat using your other leg.

Notes:
• Be dynamic and react to the ball's movements.
• Keep your arms by your side or across your lap to reduce your arm movements and encourage pelvic reactions.
• Remember to look straight ahead.
• Keep your pelvis level.

Progressions:
• When you can perform this exercise with good control whilst maintaining correct postural alignment attempt to perform it with your eyes closed.
• Once this exercise becomes easy move on to Seated Straight Leg Lifts Level 2.

Swiss Ball Exercises

Effective Swiss Ball Training

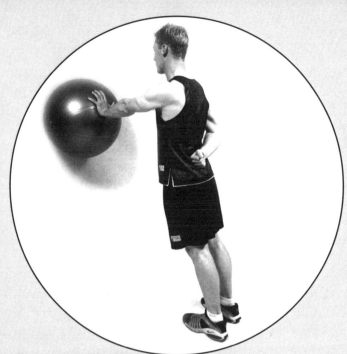

Main Focus of this Exercise:
• Shoulder and scapular mobility.
• Shoulder muscular control.

How to perform this Exercise:
• Stand with the ball positioned at shoulder height against a wall.
• Lean against the ball keeping your arms and spine straight.
• Move the ball in all four directions as far as you can using only your shoulder.
• Aim for a maximum range of motion without bending your spine, knees or arms.

Notes:
• Be sure to maintain a neutral spinal alignment.
• Remember to keep your arms straight.
• As you progress this exercise, be increasingly aware of maintaining your spine in a neutral position.

Progressions:
• If you are using this exercise as part of your rehabilitation from a shoulder injury be sure to consult your physician before attempting to progress this to more challenging exercise.
• Once you have achieved good control and a large range of motion, try to lower the ball down the wall and move your feet further away from the wall.

Trunk Rotations - Level 1

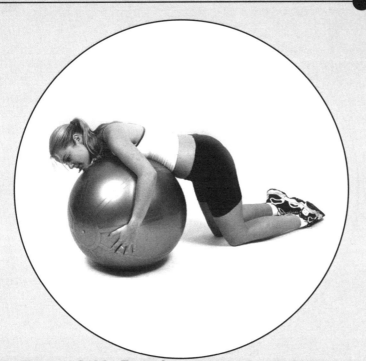

Main Focus of this Exercise:
• Mid to upper thoracic spine rotational mobility.
• Core control.
• Upper spine muscular flexibility.

How to perform this Exercise:
• Kneel in front of the ball with your knees at shoulder width apart and your chest and chin resting on top of the ball.
• Roll the ball from side to side rotating your upper body.
• Aim for a maximal range of motion whilst keeping both knees on the ground.

Notes:
• Keep a space between the ball and your thighs.
• Keep your neck relaxed and your chest on top of the ball.

Progressions:
• When you achieve your maximal range of motion with your knees at shoulder width apart, bring your knees closer together to create a narrower base of support.

Trunk Rotations - Level 2

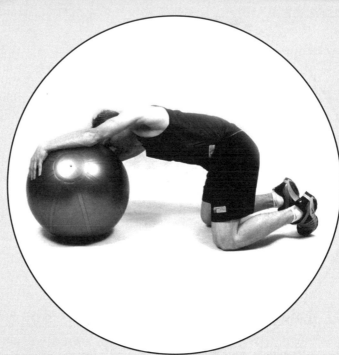

Main Focus of this Exercise::
• Whole spine rotational mobility.
• Core control.
• Spinal muscular flexibility.

How to perform this Exercise:
• Kneel in front of the ball with your arms outstretched and hands at shoulder width on top of the ball.
• Roll the ball from side to side rotating your body.
• Aim for a maximal range of motion whilst keeping both knees on the ground.

Notes:
• Keep a space between the ball and your thighs.
• Keep your neck and upper back in a neutral position.
• Keep your knees directly underneath your hips.

Progressions:
• When you achieve your maximal range of motion with your knees at shoulder width apart, bring your knees closer together to create a narrower base of support.

Prone Leg Abduction

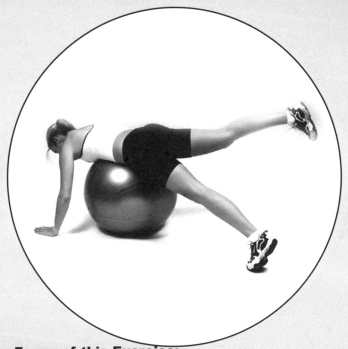

Main Focus of this Exercise:
• Gluteal, hip and spinal strength.
• Hip joint mobility.

How to perform this Exercise:
• Lie on your stomach with the ball placed underneath your hips.
• Support yourself with your arms shoulder width apart and your feet on the ground.
• Slowly lift up one straight leg and move it out to the side.
• Return your leg to the ground and repeat using your other leg.
• Aim for a maximum range of motion.

Notes:
• Keep your legs straight.
• Maintain your spine in a slightly flexed or neutral position but avoid arching it when you lift your leg.

Progressions:
• This exercise can be made more challenging by combining it with the Prone Alternate Arm Lift exercise.

Swiss Ball Exercises

Effective Swiss Ball Training

Pelvic Lift with Support

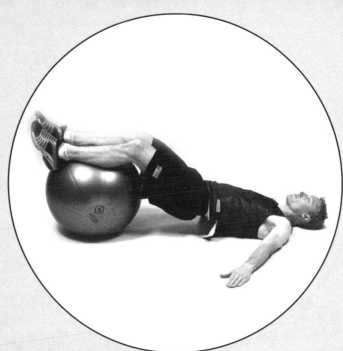

Main Focus of this Exercise:
• Gluteal, spinal and hamstring strength.
• Gluteal tone.
• Core control.

How to perform this Exercise:
• Lie on your back with the ball placed underneath your knees.
• With your knees shoulder width apart, outstretch your arms on the ground.
• Slowly lift your pelvis off the ground.
• Return your pelvis to the ground and repeat.

Notes:
• Keep your spine in a neutral position.
• This exercise may not be suitable if you have any spinal pain or have had a recent spinal injury.

Progressions:
• To make this exercise more challenging bring your feet closer together.
• When this exercise becomes easy move onto Pelvic Lifts - Level 1.

Ab Squeeze

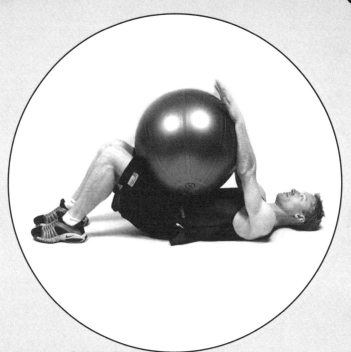

Main Focus of this Exercise:
• Abdominal, hip and arm strength.
How to perform this Exercise:
• Lie on your back with the ball on your stomach.
• Hold the ball between your arms and legs.
• Using your abdominal muscles squeeze the ball by trying to curl up your body.
• Hold this for 5 seconds.
• Relax and repeat.
Notes:
• Think of pulling your lower ribs towards your thighs.
• Keep your neck relaxed.
• Keep looking up at the roof and be sure to keep breathing.
Progressions:
• The progression of this exercise is to simply squeeze harder or increase the amount of time you hold the contraction.

Swiss Ball Exercises

Effective Swiss Ball Training

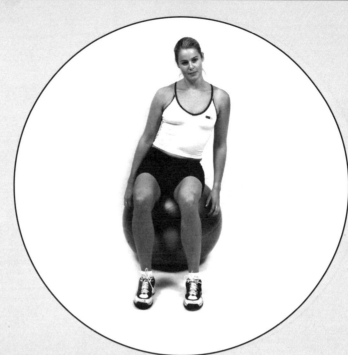

Main Focus of this Exercise:
• Core control.
• Abdominal tone.
• Balance.

How to perform this Exercise:
• Sit on the ball with your feet shoulder width apart.
• Shift your body to the left and right on the ball.
• As you improve, bring your feet closer together or try lifting a leg whilst moving.

Notes:
• React to the movements of the ball.
• Minimise your arm movements.
• Maintain a neutral pelvic alignment.
• Look straight ahead.

Lying Side Rolls - Level 1

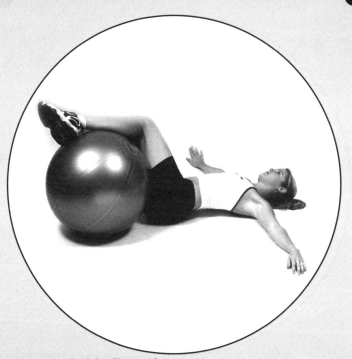

Main Focus of this Exercise:
• Oblique strength and tone.
• Core control.
• Spinal mobility.

How to perform this Exercise:
• Lie on your back with the ball placed underneath your knees and your arms outstretched to the sides.
• Roll your legs from side to side keeping your shoulders on the ground at all times.

Notes:
• Keep your shoulders on the ground and keep looking towards the roof.

Progressions:
• When you can perform this exercise with a good range of motion and control move onto Lying Side Rolls – Level 2.

Swiss Ball Exercises

Effective Swiss Ball Training

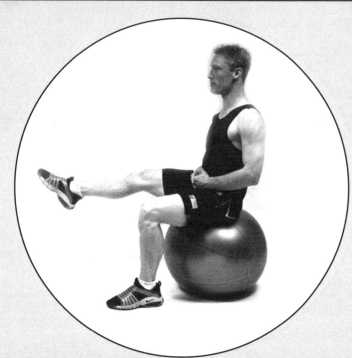

Main Focus of this Exercise:
• Core control.
• Abdominal tone.
• Dynamic balance.

How to perform this Exercise:
• Sit on the ball.
• Lift one leg off the ground.
• Straighten out your leg.
• Move your straight leg out to the side whilst maintaining a level pelvis and your balance on the ball.
• Return your leg to its starting position and then to the ground.
• Repeat using your other leg.

Notes:
• Be dynamic and react to the ball's movements.
• Keep your arms by your side or across your lap to reduce your arm movements and encourage pelvic reactions.
• Remember to look straight ahead.
• Keep your pelvis level.

Progressions:
• To make this exercise more challenging close your eyes or place your grounded foot on a pillow or cushion.

Shoulder Stability Exercise

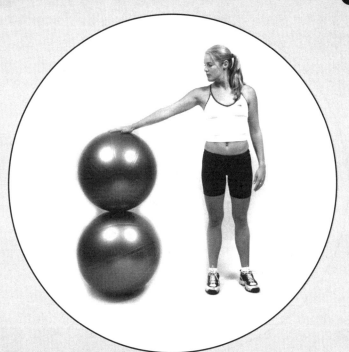

Main Focus of this Exercise:
• Shoulder and scapula stability and muscular control.
• Shoulder proprioception

How to perform this Exercise:
• Place one small ball on top of another and whilst standing, use your hand to push down on top of the balls.
• Maintain enough pressure to keep the balls together without unbalancing them.
• Try to increase the pressure you apply without unbalancing the balls.

Notes:
• Keep your shoulders back and arms straight.
• Maintain neutral spinal alignment.
• Use balls that are such a size to come up to just above waist level when on top of each other.

Progressions:
• As this exercise gets easier increase the amount of pressure you apply to the top ball and/or close your eyes.

Swiss Ball Exercises

Effective Swiss Ball Training

Ab Crunches Seated

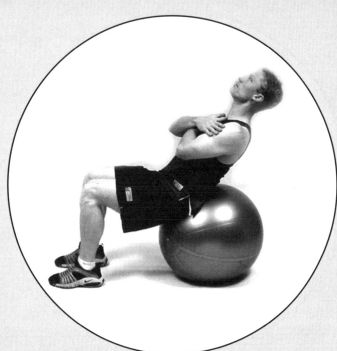

Main Focus of this Exercise:
• Abdominal strength and tone.
• Core control.
• Dynamic balance.

How to perform this Exercise:
• Sit so that you are leaning back with the ball placed under your lumbar spine.
• Slowly lift your trunk up towards the roof to a near seated position.
• Lean back down to your starting position.
• Repeat exercise slowly with good control and maintain a neutral spine.

Notes:
• Always keep your neck in a neutral position to avoid using your neck muscles.
• This exercise may not be suitable if you have had a recent spinal injury or a history of spinal disc injury.

Progressions:
• The progression of this exercise is to increase your leverage length by putting your hands to your ears.
• Once that becomes easy or you can comfortably perform 3 sets of 15 repetitions, try straightening your arms out above your head to further increase your leverage length.

Wall Ball Squats - 2 Legs

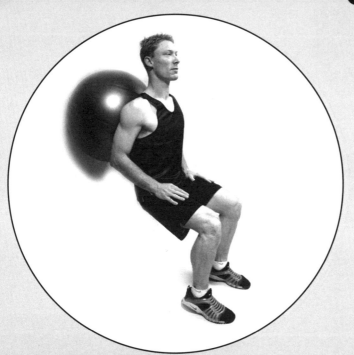

Main Focus of this Exercise:
• Leg, hip and gluteal strength and tone.
How to perform this Exercise:
• Place the ball against a wall and lean your mid back against it.
• With your feet at shoulder width apart, slowly squat down until your hips are at the same level as your knees so your thighs are parallel with the floor.
• Stand back upright slowly and repeat.
Notes:
• Keep your spine in a neutral position at all times.
• Remember to only go down to the point where you are comfortable and only ever go low enough so your thighs are parallel with the floor.
Progressions:
• When you can perform 3 sets of 12 repetitions of this exercise comfortably progress onto Wall Ball Squats – 1 Leg.

Wall Ball Calf Raises - 2 Legs

Swiss Ball Exercises

Effective Swiss Ball Training

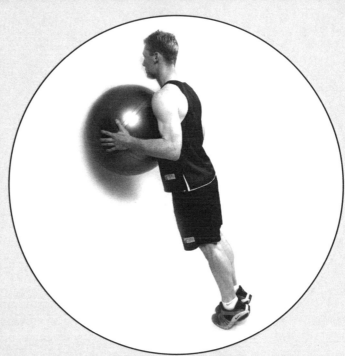

Main Focus of this Exercise:
• Calf strength and tone.

How to perform this Exercise:
• Place the ball against a wall and lean against the ball with your lower chest.
• Separate your feet slightly and raise yourself up onto your toes.
• Lower and repeat.

Notes:
• Keep your spine in neutral alignment at all times.

Progressions:
• This exercise can be progressed by lowering the height of the ball on the wall to increase the range of motion and angle you must push against.
• When this exercise becomes easy progress to Wall Ball Calf Raises – 1 Leg.

Prone Back Extension - Level 1

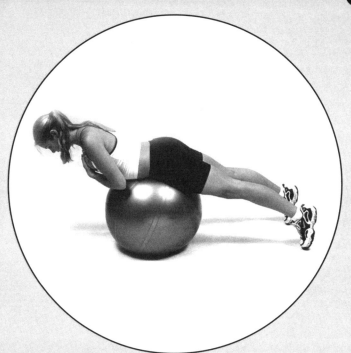

Main Focus of this Exercise:
• Lumbar spine extension mobility and strength.

How to perform this Exercise:
• Lie on your stomach with the ball placed under your hips starting with your upper body curled forward over the ball.
• Cross your arms across your chest.
• Slowly lift and extend your upper body until your spine is in a neutral alignment.
• Slowly return to flexed forward position and repeat slowly.

Notes:
• Keep looking at the ground and keep your neck in a neutral position.
• Separate your feet to maintain stability.

Progressions:
• To make this exercise more challenging, place your hands behind your head.
• To make it even more challenging straighten your arms out in front of you.

Swiss Ball Exercises

Effective Swiss Ball Training

Lying Side Rolls - Level 2

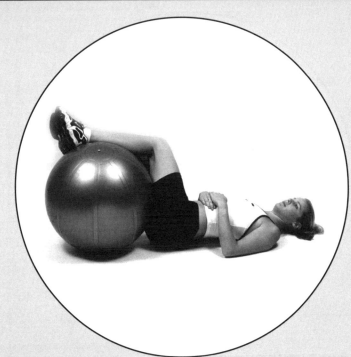

Main Focus of this Exercise:
• Oblique strength and tone.
• Core control.
• Spinal mobility.

How to perform this Exercise:
• Lie on your back with the ball placed underneath your knees and your elbows by your side and your hands on your stomach.
• Roll your legs from side to side keeping your shoulders on the ground at all times.

Notes:
• Keep your shoulders on the ground and keep looking towards the roof.

Progressions:
• When you can perform this exercise with a good range of motion and control move onto Lying Side Rolls – Level 3.

Supine Bridge

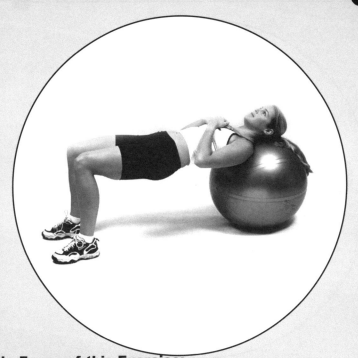

Main Focus of this Exercise:
• Spinal, gluteal and quadriceps strength.
• Core control.

How to perform this Exercise:
• Sit on the ball and slowly walk your feet forward whilst leaning back onto the ball.
• Do this until your head and neck are supported on the ball and your spine is in a neutral alignment.
• Hold this position with your spine in a neutral alignment for 3 - 5 seconds before slowly returning to the starting position.

Notes:
• Keep your spine in a neutral alignment to avoid hyperextension.
• Keep your head and neck supported on the ball.
• Keep your knees placed directly over your heels.

Progressions:
• Once you can perform 2 sets of 10 repetitions of this exercise holding the position for 10 seconds each time try to move onto Supine Bridge with Dips.

Prone Walk Forwards

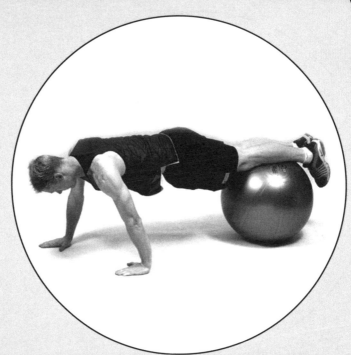

Main Focus of this Exercise:
• Shoulder, arm and upper back strength.
• Shoulder and core muscular control.

How to perform this Exercise:
• Kneel in front of the ball.
• Roll forward over the top of the ball and slowly walk forward using your hands.
• Walk back to the initial kneeling point and repeat.

Notes:
• Keep your elbows straight and walk slowly.
• If you have wrist or hand problems try to make a fist and walk on your knuckles.

Progressions:
• As you improve, increase the amount of time spent on one hand or walk further out until the tips of your toes are on the ball.
• Once you can perform this exercise with ease move onto Push Ups – Feet on Ball – Level 1.

Reverse Curls with Ball

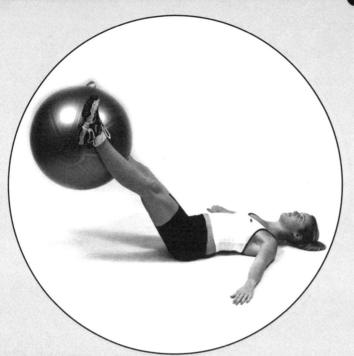

Main Focus of this Exercise:
• Abdominal strength and tone.
• Core control.

How to perform this Exercise:
• Lie on your back with the ball placed between your legs and your hands by your side.
• Slowly bring your knees towards your chest so that the ball is off the ground.
• Straighten your legs out as far as you can lowering the ball, whilst maintaining pressure between your lumbar spine and the ground.
• Rest the ball on the ground between sets.

Notes:
• Keep your movements slow and controlled.
• Maintain pressure between your lumbar spine and the ground at all times.
• If your back starts to arch then reduce how far you straighten your legs out.
• Keep breathing throughout the exercise.

Progressions:
• The progression of this exercise is to be able to straighten your legs out further whilst still maintaining good pressure between your lumbar spine and the ground.
• Once you can achieve this place your arms across your stomach and repeat the exercise.
• You may need to reduce how far you straighten your legs again until you can achieve good control.

Swiss Ball Exercises

Effective Swiss Ball Training

Pelvic Lifts - Level 1

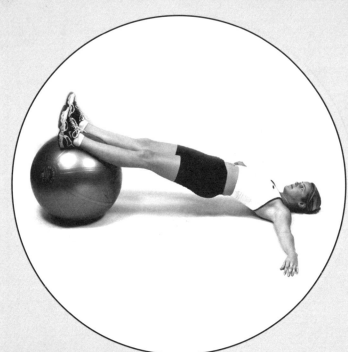

Main Focus of this Exercise:
• Gluteal, spinal and hamstring strength.
• Gluteal tone.
• Core control.

How to perform this Exercise:
• Lie on your back with the ball placed underneath your feet.
• With your feet shoulder width apart and your arms outstretched on the ground, slowly lift your pelvis so that your spine is in a neutral alignment.
• Return your pelvis to the ground and repeat.

Notes:
• Maintain good spinal alignment to avoid hyperextension.
• This exercise may not be suitable if you have had a recent spinal injury.

Progressions:
• You can make this exercise more challenging by bringing your feet closer together on the ball.
• When you can perform 3 sets of 10 repetitions of this exercise holding each repetition for 5 seconds comfortably move onto Pelvic Lifts – Level 2.

Supine Bridge with Dips

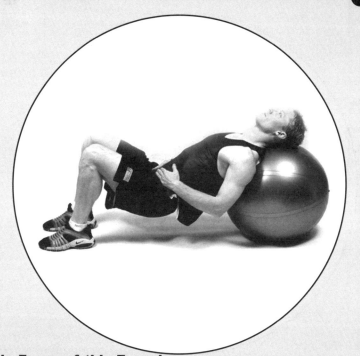

Main Focus of this Exercise:
• Spinal, gluteal and quadriceps strength.
• Core control.
• Gluteal tone.

How to perform this Exercise:
• Sit on the ball and slowly walk your feet forward whilst leaning back onto the ball.
• Do this until your head and neck are supported on the ball and your spine is in a neutral alignment.
• Slowly lower your buttocks down towards the ground without rolling forward on the ball.
• Lift your pelvis back up to a neutral spinal alignment.
• When you have completed several repetitions slowly return to the seated starting position.

Notes:
• When you lift your pelvis back up be sure to only go to a point where your spine is in a neutral alignment to avoid hyperextension.
• Keep your head and neck supported on the ball.

Progressions:
• Once you can perform 2 sets of 12 repetitions of this exercise try combining it with the Supine Bridge with Alternate Leg Lift exercise for a great challenge.

Swiss Ball Exercises

Effective Swiss Ball Training

Baby Crawl

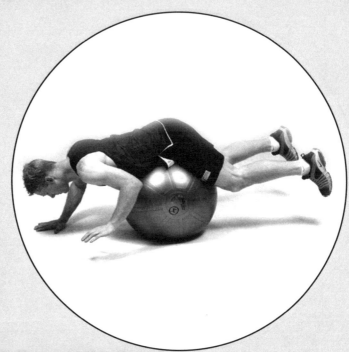

Main Focus of this Exercise:
• Core control.
• Abdominal strength and tone.

How to perform this Exercise:
• Lie on your stomach with your hands on legs in contact with the floor.
• Adjust your body position so as you can lift both feet and one hand off the ground leaving you balancing on one hand.
• Balance in this position for 5 seconds before changing hands.
• Balance in this position for 5 seconds before changing to one foot with neither hand in contact with the ground.
• Balance in this position for 5 seconds before switching to the other foot.

Notes:
• Keep your head looking down at the ground to avoid extending your neck.

Progressions:
• This exercise can be made more challenging by spending longer on each limb before switching to the next limb.
• It can also be made more difficult be closing your eyes whilst trying to balance.

Lying Side Rolls - Level 3

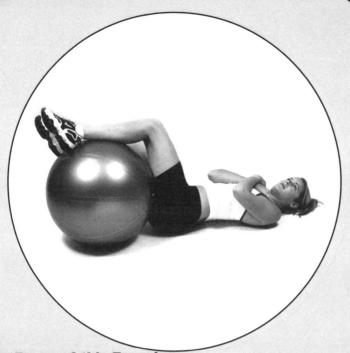

Main Focus of this Exercise:
• Oblique strength and tone.
• Core control.
• Spinal mobility.

How to perform this Exercise:
• Lie on your back with the ball placed underneath your knees and your arms crossed across your chest so that your elbows are off the ground.
• Roll your legs from side to side keeping your shoulders on the ground at all times.

Notes:
• Keep your shoulders on the ground and keep looking towards the roof.

Prone Roll Forwards

Swiss Ball Exercises

Effective Swiss Ball Training

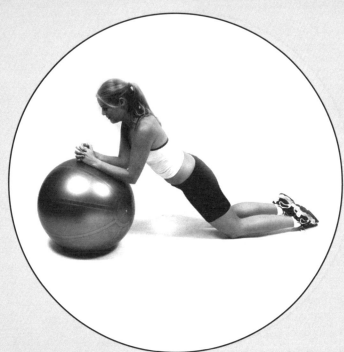

Main Focus of this Exercise:
• Core and chest strength.
• Shoulder stability.
• Abdominal strength and tone.

How to perform this Exercise:
• Kneel In front of the ball with your arms outstretched and fists together on top of the ball.
• Lean your body forward and roll the ball forward whilst pushing your fists down into the ball.

Notes:
• Maintain a neutral spinal alignment to avoid hyperextension of your spine.

Progressions:
• As you improve, roll further forward allowing your buttocks to drop down towards the ground but whilst still maintaining a neutral spinal alignment.

Prone Back Extension - Level 2

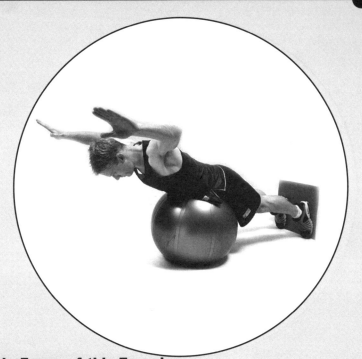

Main Focus of this Exercise:
• Spinal extension mobility.
• Spinal strength.
• Gluteal strength and tone.

How to perform this Exercise:
• Lie on your stomach with the ball placed underneath your hips.
• Place your legs out straight with your feet against the base of a wall.
• Allow your upper body to curl forward over the ball.
• Lift your upper body until your spine is in a neutral alignment with your arms outstretched above your head.
• Slowly return to your original curled forward position and repeat.

Notes:
• Keep your face looking down and neck in a neutral alignment.
• Separate your feet to maintain stability.

Swiss Ball Exercises

Effective Swiss Ball Training

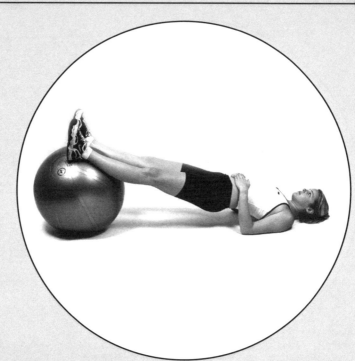

Main Focus of this Exercise:
• Gluteal, spinal and hamstring strength.
• Gluteal tone.
• Core control.

How to perform this Exercise:
• Lie on your back with the ball placed underneath your feet.
• With your feet shoulder width apart, place your elbows on the ground and your arms crossed across your stomach.
• Slowly lift your pelvis so that your spine is in a neutral alignment.
• Return your pelvis to the ground and repeat.

Notes:
• Maintain good spinal alignment to avoid hyperextension.
• This exercise may not be suitable if you have had a recent spinal injury.

Progressions:
• You can make this exercise more challenging by bringing your feet closer together on the ball.
• When you can perform 3 sets of 10 repetitions of this exercise holding each repetition for 5 seconds comfortably move onto Pelvic Lifts – Level 3.

Wall Ball Calf Raises - 1 Leg

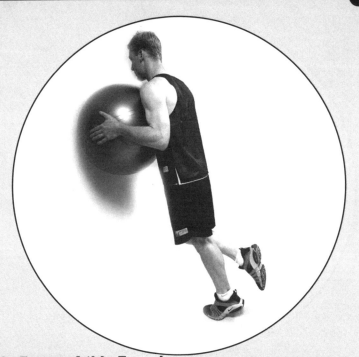

Main Focus of this Exercise:
• Calf strength and muscular balance.
• Dynamic balance.

How to perform this Exercise:
• Place the ball against a wall and lean against the ball with your lower chest.
• Lift one leg off ground and using your supporting leg, raise yourself up onto your toes.
• Lower and repeat several times before repeating with the other leg.

Notes:
• Keep your spine in a neutral alignment at all times.

Progressions:
• This exercise can be made more difficult by lowering the height of the ball on the wall to increase the range of motion and the angle you must push against.

Prone Tuck Ins

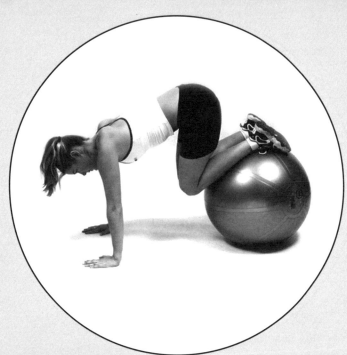

Main Focus of this Exercise:
• Shoulder, arm and upper back strength.
• Abdominal strength and tone.
• Lumbar spine flexion mobility.

How to perform this Exercise:
• Kneel in front of the ball.
• Roll forward over the top of the ball and slowly walk forward using your hands until the ball is under your lower legs or your feet.
• Bring your knees and the ball up towards your chest until your body is in a curled up position.
• Slowly take your knees and the ball back until your legs are straight again.
• Repeat this 'Tuck In' several times before walking back to the initial kneeling point and repeat.

Notes:
• Maintain good postural alignment to avoid hyperextension of your lumbar spine.

Progressions:
• When you can perform 3 sets of 10 Tuck Ins of this exercise with good control move onto Prone Oblique Tuck Ins.

Windscreen Wipers

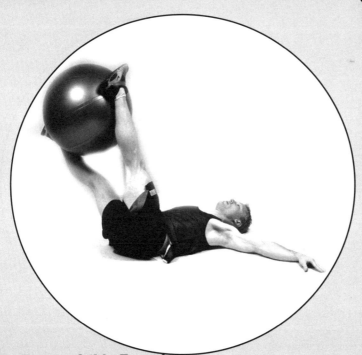

Main Focus of this Exercise:
• Adductor muscle strength and tone.
• Obliques muscular strength and tone.
• Core control.

How to perform this Exercise:
• Lie on your back with the ball placed between your feet and your arms outstretched to the side..
• Grip the ball between your feet and lift it up above your pelvis so that your legs are nearly straight.
• Rotate your legs from side to side as far as you can go comfortably.

Notes:
• Keep your shoulders in contact with the ground at all times.
• Keep breathing throughout the exercise.

Swiss Ball Exercises

Effective Swiss Ball Training

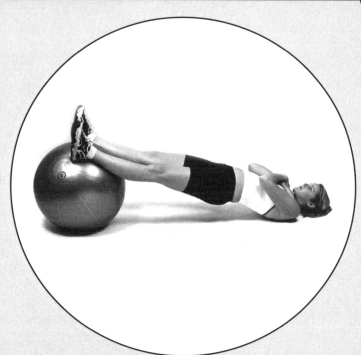

Main Focus of this Exercise:
• Gluteal, spinal and hamstring strength.
• Gluteal tone.
• Core control.

How to perform this Exercise:
• Lie on your back with the ball placed underneath your feet.
• With your feet shoulder width apart cross your arms across your chest so that your elbows are off the ground.
• Slowly lift your pelvis so that your spine is in a neutral alignment.
• Return your pelvis to the ground and repeat.

Notes:
• Maintain good spinal alignment to avoid hyperextension.
• This exercise may not be suitable if you have had a recent spinal injury.

Progressions:
• You can make this exercise more challenging by bringing your feet closer together on the ball.
• When you can perform 3 sets of 10 repetitions of this exercise holding each repetition for 5 seconds comfortably try to maintain the elevated position whilst slowly shifting the ball from side to side.

Side Lifts on Ball - Level 1

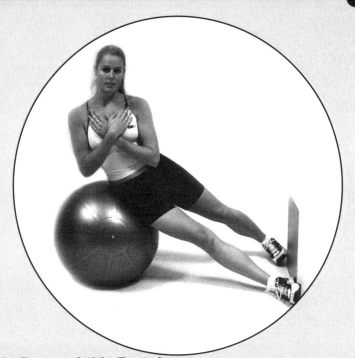

Main Focus of this Exercise:
• Oblique abdominal strength and tone.
• Lateral spinal muscular strength and tone.

How to perform this Exercise:
• Start by sitting sideways on the ball so that one hip is placed directly on top of the ball.
• Separate your feet out wide and place them against the base of a wall.
• Cross your arms across your chest and slowly lower your upper down over the ball.
• Lift your body up to its original elevated position.
• When you have completed several repetitions on one hip swap over to your other hip and repeat.

Notes:
• Maintain neutral spinal alignment

Progressions:
• This exercise can be made more challenging by moving the ball further down your hip towards your leg so as to increase the range of motion you can move through and the amount of your body which is unsupported.
• When you can perform 3 sets of 12 repetitions on each side move onto Side Lifts on Ball – Level 2.

Swiss Ball Exercises

Effective Swiss Ball Training

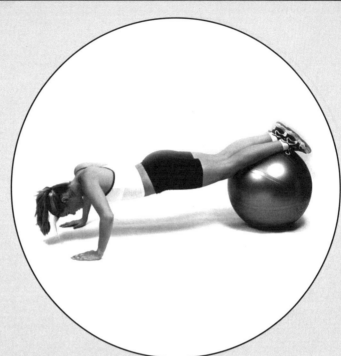

Main Focus of this Exercise:
• Shoulder, chest and arm strength and tone.
• Shoulder stability.
• Core control.

How to perform this Exercise:
• Start this exercise with a Prone Walk Forward and when you get to a comfortable position lower your chest down towards the ground until your chin nearly touches the ground.
• Repeat this several times before walking back to your initial position.

Notes:
• Keep a neutral spinal alignment.
• Look at a spot just in front of an imaginary line between your thumbs.
• Lowering yourself all the way to the ground is more important than how many repetitions you can perform.
• Remember to keep your back straight and lower your whole body rather than bending at the hips.

Progressions:
• The progression of this exercise is to walk further out initially until you have the tips of your toes on the ball.
• When you can complete 3 sets of 12 push ups try to progress to Push Ups Hands on Ball.

Prone Oblique Tuck Ins

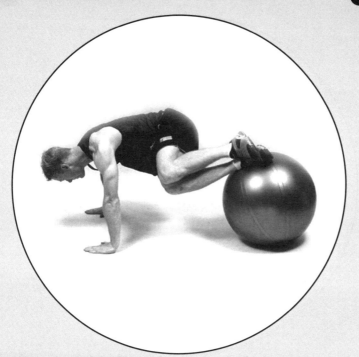

Main Focus of this Exercise:
• Shoulder, arm and upper back strength.
• Shoulder stability.
• Abdominal and oblique strength and tone.
• Lumbar spine flexion and rotation mobility.

How to perform this Exercise:
• Kneel in front of the ball.
• This exercise starts with a Prone Walk Forward until the ball is at least past your knees.
• In this position, bring your knees and the ball up to towards your chest whilst rotating your hips and legs to one side to finish in a curled and rotated position.
• Slowly take your knees and the ball back until your legs are straight again.
• Repeat this on the other side of your body.

Notes:
• This exercise may not be suitable if you have a recent spinal injury or a chronic spinal condition.
• Remember to keep your head looking down towards the ground.

Progressions:
• The progression of this exercise is to walk further out initially until you have your toes on the ball.

Swiss Ball Exercises

Effective Swiss Ball Training

Ball Dips - Hands on Ball

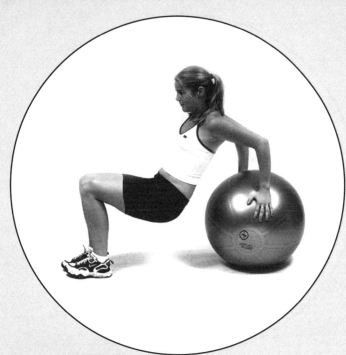

Main Focus of this Exercise:
• Arm strength and tone.
• Abdominal strength.

How to perform this Exercise:
• Sit on the ball and place your hands on the ball just behind your buttocks with your fingers facing behind you.
• Place your feet flat on the ground shoulder width apart a small distance in front of you.
• Move forward taking your body weight on your hands so your buttocks is off the ball.
• Slowly lower your buttocks down towards the ground allowing your elbows to bend as you go down.
• Push yourself back up until your arms are straight again and repeat.

Notes:
• Remember to look straight ahead at all times.
• A full range of motion is important before attempting to progress this exercise.

Progressions:
• To make this exercise more challenging you can move your feet closer together and further from the ball until your legs are straight.
• When you can perform 3 sets of 10 repetitions of this exercise try Ball Dips Feet on Ball.

Ball Dips - Feet on Ball - Level 1

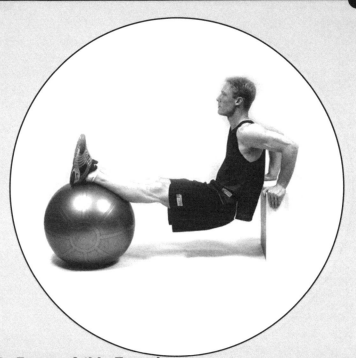

Main Focus of this Exercise:
• Arm strength and tone.
• Abdominal strength.

How to perform this Exercise:
• Sit on a bench and place your hands on the edge of the bench next to you.
• Place your lower legs shoulder width apart on top of the ball.
• Move forward taking your body weight on your hands so your buttocks is off the bench.
• Slowly lower your buttocks down towards the ground allowing your elbows to bend as you go down.
• Push yourself back up until your arms are straight again and repeat.

Notes:
• Remember to look straight ahead at all times.
• A full range of motion is important before attempting to progress this exercise.

Progressions:
• To make this exercise more challenging you can move your legs closer together and move the ball further away from you until your legs are straight.
• When you can perform 3 sets of 10 repetitions of this exercise try Ball Dips Feet on Ball – Level 2.

Swiss Ball Exercises

Effective Swiss Ball Training

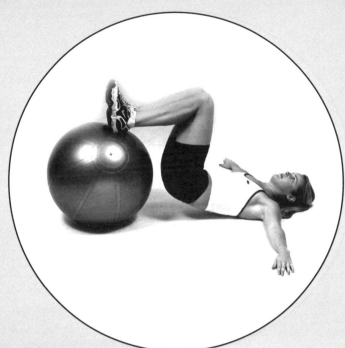

Main Focus of this Exercise:
• Gluteal, spinal and hamstring strength.
• Gluteal tone.
• Core control.

How to perform this Exercise:
• Start by performing a Pelvic Lift – Level 1.
• When you are in a position with your spine off the ground slowly bring your knees towards your chest.
• Return your legs to a straight position and lower your buttocks back down to the ground.

Notes:
• Try to keep your buttocks off the ground throughout the tuck in.

Progressions:
• To make this exercise more challenging move your legs closer together or move the ball further away from you until your heels are on top of the ball.
• When you can perform 3 sets of 10 repetitions of this exercise try Pelvic Lifts with Tuck Ins – Level 2.

Push Ups Hand on Ball

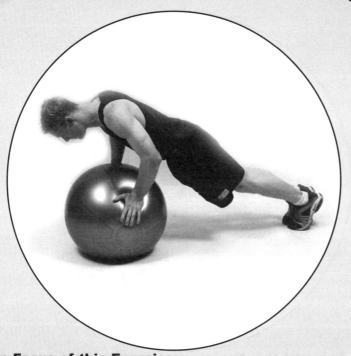

Main Focus of this Exercise:
• Shoulder stability.
• Chest and arm strength.
• Shoulder proprioception.
• Core control.

How to perform this Exercise:
• Start in a lying position with the ball placed underneath your chest.
• Place your hands on top of the ball at shoulder width apart and push your body up until your elbows are nearly straight.
• Lower your chest back down until it nearly touches the ball and repeat.

Notes:
• Keep hands pointed 45 degrees away from you.
• Keep your spine in a neutral alignment.
• Keep your feet together.
• Keep your elbows slightly bent when you have pushed up fully.

Progressions:
• When you can perform 3 sets of 10 repetitions of this exercise try Push Ups Feet on Ball – Level 2.

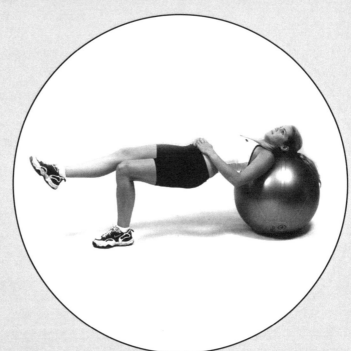

Main Focus of this Exercise:
• Spinal, gluteal, hamstring and quadriceps strength.
• Core control.
• Hip, ankle and knee stability.

How to perform this Exercise:
• Start by performing a Supine Bridge exercise.
• When you are in the bridge position straighten and lift one leg whilst maintaining neutral pelvic alignment.
• As you improve, increase the amount of time spent on each leg.

Notes:
• Keep your spine in a neutral alignment to avoid hyperextension..
• Be sure to keep your head and neck supported on the ball at all times.
• Keep your knees directly over your heels.

Progressions:
• To make this exercise more challenging try spending longer on each leg before changing or perform this exercise with your eyes closed.

Pelvic Lifts with tuck ins - Level 2

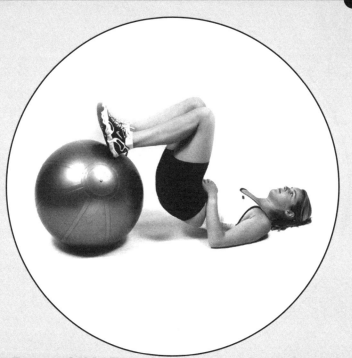

Main Focus of this Exercise:
• Gluteal, spinal and hamstring strength.
• Gluteal tone.
• Core control.

How to perform this Exercise:
• Start by performing a Pelvic Lift – Level 2.
• When you are in a position with your spine off the ground slowly bring your knees towards your chest.
• Return your legs to a straight position and lower your buttocks back down to the ground.

Notes:
• Try to keep your buttocks off the ground throughout the tuck in.

Progressions:
• When you can perform 3 sets of 10 repetitions of this exercise try Pelvic Lifts with Tuck Ins – Level 3.

Swiss Ball Exercises

Effective Swiss Ball Training

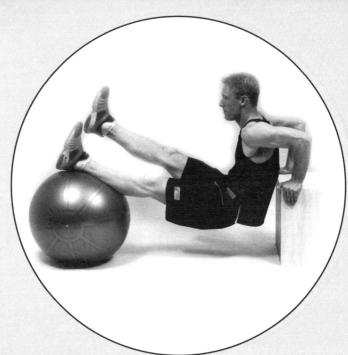

Main Focus of this Exercise:
• Arm strength and tone.
• Abdominal strength.

How to perform this Exercise:
• Start by getting into position for Ball Dips Feet on Ball – Level 1.
• When you are in position lift one leg off the ball and hold it in the air whilst you slowly lower your buttocks down towards the ground allowing your elbows to bend as you go down.
• Push yourself back up until your arms are straight again.
• Repeat this several times before performing another set on your alternate leg.

Notes:
• Remember to look straight ahead at all times.
• A full range of motion is important before attempting to progress this exercise.

Push Ups with Feet on Ball - Level 2

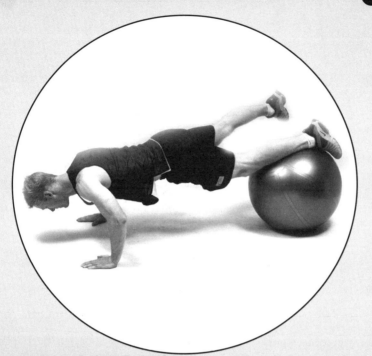

Main Focus of this Exercise:
• Shoulder, chest and arm strength and tone.
• Shoulder stability.
• Core control.

How to perform this Exercise:
• Start this exercise with a Prone Walk Forward.
• When you have walked forward to a comfortable position lift one leg off the ball and hold it in the air.
• While holding this leg in the air, lower your chest down towards the ground until your chin nearly touches the ground.
• Repeat this several times before performing another set on your alternate leg.

Notes:
• Keep a neutral spinal alignment.
• Look at a spot just in front of an imaginary line between your thumbs.
• Lowering yourself all the way to the ground is more important than how many repetitions you can perform.
• Remember to keep your back straight and lower your whole body rather than bending at the hips.

Progressions:
• The progression of this exercise is to walk further out initially until you have the tips of your toes on the ball.
• When you can complete 3 sets of 12 push ups try to progress to Push Ups Hands on Ball.

Swiss Ball Exercises

Effective Swiss Ball Training

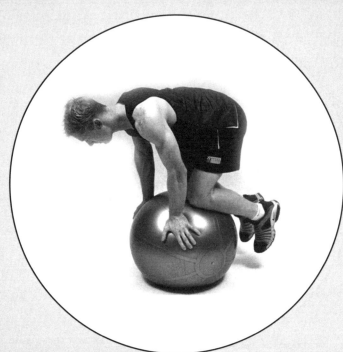

Main Focus of this Exercise:
• Balance.
• Core control.
• Spinal and abdominal strength.

How to perform this Exercise:
• Start by standing behind the ball with your hands shoulder width apart on top of the ball.
• Bend your knees forward until they touch the ball.
• Slowly lean forward pushing yourself up onto your toes.
• Continue to lean forward until your toes come off the ground and you are balancing on your hands and knees on the ball.
• React to every movement the ball makes.
• To finish slowly roll back until your feet touch the ground.

Notes:
• This is an advanced exercise. Attempt it at your own risk.
• When attempting this exercise at first it is best to try it with a partner next to you to assist you when you become unbalanced.
• It is also a good idea to place several cushions or soft mats around you at first until you are confident balancing on the ball.

Progressions:
• When you can perform this exercise comfortably for over 30 seconds try to attempt Kneeling on Ball – Level 2.

Pelvic Lift with One Leg Lift

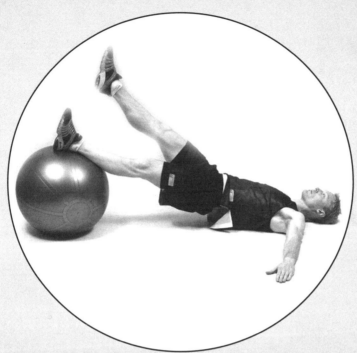

Main Focus of this Exercise:
• Gluteal, spinal and hamstring strength.
• Gluteal tone.
• Core control.

How to perform this Exercise:
• Start by performing a Pelvic Lift – Level 3.
• When you are in a position with your spine lifted off the ground try to lift one leg off the ball whilst maintaining a neutral pelvic alignment.
• Return your leg to the ball and your pelvis to the ground and repeat on your alternate leg.

Notes:
• Maintain good spinal alignment to avoid hyperextension.
• This exercise may not be suitable if you have had a recent spinal injury.

Progressions:
• When you can perform 3 sets of 10 repetitions of this exercise holding each repetition for 5 seconds comfortably try to perform Pelvic Lifts with Tuck Ins - Level 3.

Swiss Ball Exercises

Effective Swiss Ball Training

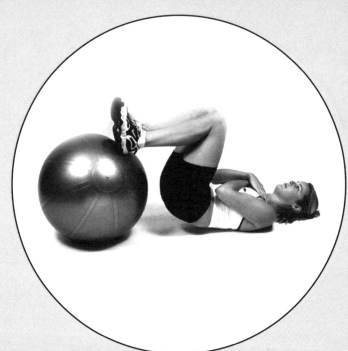

Main Focus of this Exercise:
• Gluteal, spinal and hamstring strength.
• Gluteal tone.
• Core control.
How to perform this Exercise:
• Start by performing a Pelvic Lift – Level 2.
• Cross your arms across your chest and when you are in a position with your spine off the ground slowly bring your knees towards your chest.
• Return your legs to a straight position and lower your buttocks back down to the ground.
Notes:
• Try to keep your buttocks off the ground throughout the tuck in.
Progressions:
• When you can perform 3 sets of 10 repetitions of this exercise try Pelvic Lifts with One Leg Tuck Ins.

Wall Ball Squat - 1 Leg

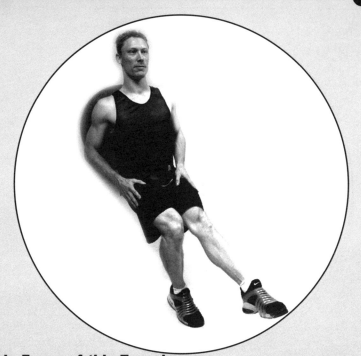

Main Focus of this Exercise:
• Leg, hip and gluteal strength and tone.
How to perform this Exercise:
• Start by leaning back with upper back against ball and ball placed against wall and feet slightly out in front at shoulder width.
• Lift one leg off the ground and slowly squat down until your thigh is parallel with the floor.
• Stand back upright and repeat on other leg.
Notes:
• Keep your spine in a neutral alignment at all times.
• Remember to only go down to the point where you're comfortable and never go lower than when your thigh is parallel with the floor.

Swiss Ball Exercises

Effective Swiss Ball Training

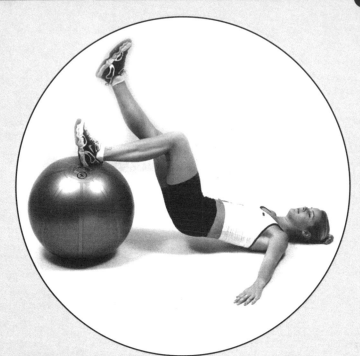

Main Focus of this Exercise:
• Gluteal, spinal and hamstring strength.
• Gluteal tone.
• Core control.

How to perform this Exercise:
• Start by performing a Pelvic Lift – Level 1.
• When you are in a position with your spine off the ground lift one leg off the ball and slowly bring your knee towards your chest.
• Return your leg to a straight position and repeat several times before lowering your buttocks back down to the ground.
• Repeat on your alternate leg.

Notes:
• Try to keep your buttocks off the ground throughout the tuck in.

Prone Walk Forwards with Alternate Arm Lifts

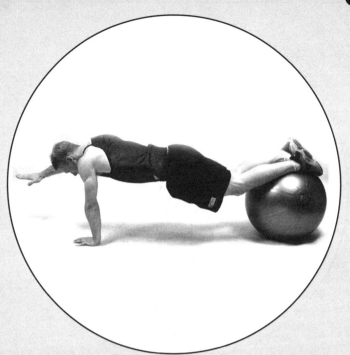

Main Focus of this Exercise:
• Shoulder, arm and upper back strength.
• Shoulder and core control.

How to perform this Exercise:
• Start by performing a Prone Walk Forward.
• Once you have walked forward to a comfortable position, lift one arm off the ground whilst still balancing on the ball.
• Return your hand to the ground and repeat using your other arm.
• When you have repeated this several times on each arm, walk back to the initial kneeling point and repeat.

Notes:
• Maintain good postural alignment avoiding rotation or hyperextension.

Progressions:
• As you improve your control of this exercise attempt it walking further forward to the point where the ball is placed under your feet.
• When this becomes easy attempt it with your eyes closed.

Swiss Ball Exercises

Effective Swiss Ball Training

Kneel on Ball - Level 2

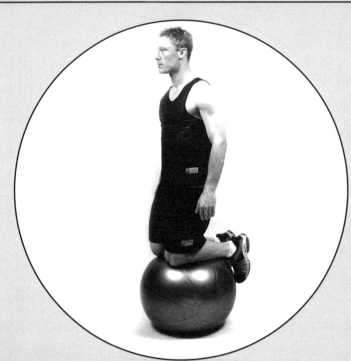

Main Focus of this Exercise:
• Balance.
• Core control.
• Spinal and abdominal strength.

How to perform this Exercise:
• Start by performing a Kneeling on Ball – Level 1.
• When you are balanced on top of the ball remove your hands and attempt to straighten your body up.
• React to every movement the ball makes.
• To finish replace your hands on the ball and slowly roll back until your feet touch the ground.

Notes:
• This is an advanced exercise. Attempt it at your own risk.
• When attempting this exercise at first it is best to try it with a partner next to you to assist you when you become unbalanced.
• It is also a good idea to place several cushions or soft mats around you at first until you are confident balancing on the ball.

Swiss Ball Stretches

Ab Stretch

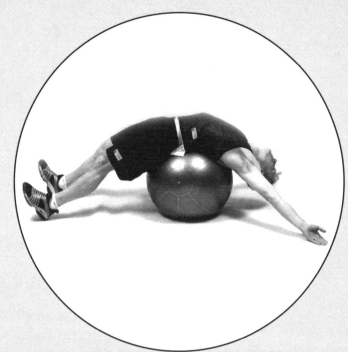

Main Focus of this Exercise:
• Increasing abdominal flexibility and spinal extension.
How to perform this Exercise:
• Lay back with ball under lower back allowing head to rest on ball.
• Only lean back as far as comfortable without pain.
• Hold this whilst breathing continually for 30 seconds.
Notes:
• This stretch may not be suitable if you have a recent spinal injury or a history of spinal disc injury.
• If you experience any pain or discomfort during this stretch cease immediately.
• Remember to continually breathe throughout this stretch.

Hip Flexor Stretch

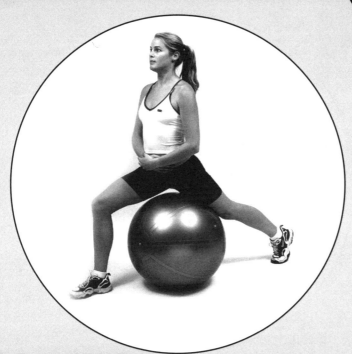

Main Focus of this Exercise:
• Increasing hip flexor flexibility.
How to perform this Exercise:
• Kneel next to the ball on one knee.
• Place the other knee over the ball.
• Lean your body back until you feel a stretch in the front of the hip of the leg on the ball.
• Hold this for 30 seconds and repeat on your other hip.
Notes:
• Only lean back as far as comfortable without experiencing any pain.

Hip Stretch

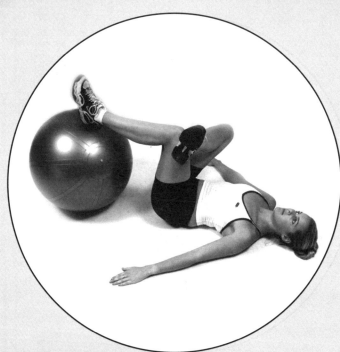

Main Focus of this Exercise:
• Increasing gluteal flexibility.

How to perform this Exercise:
• Lie on your back with one leg straight and your foot placed on top of the ball.
• Place the foot of your opposite leg across your thigh just above your knee.
• Draw the ball towards you until you feel a stretch in the buttocks of the leg which is not on the ball.
• Hold this for 30 seconds and repeat using your other leg.

Notes:
• This stretch may not be suitable if you have a recent knee injury or experience any pain in your knee.
• Only draw the ball back as far as comfortable without experiencing any pain.

Kneeling Hamstring Stretch

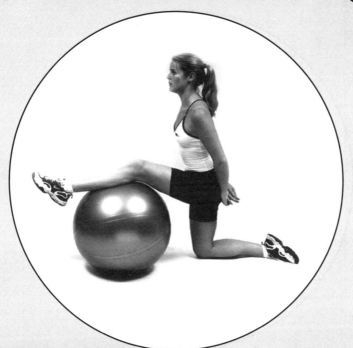

Main Focus of this Exercise:
• Increasing hamstring flexibility.

How to perform this Exercise:
• Kneel on one leg next to the ball with your other leg placed over the top of the ball.
• Allow your leg on the ball to bend at the knee slightly and slowly lean your body forward until you feel stretch at mid point of hamstrings muscle.
• Hold this for 30 seconds and repeat using your other leg.

Notes:
• Only lean forward as far as comfortable without experiencing any pain.

Spinal Flexion Stretch

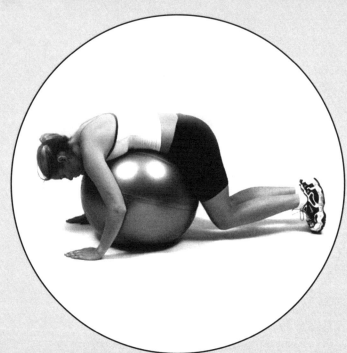

Main Focus of this Exercise:
• Increasing spinal flexion.
How to perform this Exercise:
• Lie on your stomach over the ball and allow your head to rest on the ball.
• Slowly rock forward and back to mobilise your spine.
Continue for 30 seconds.
Notes:
• Remember to continually breathe throughout this stretch.

Calf Stretch

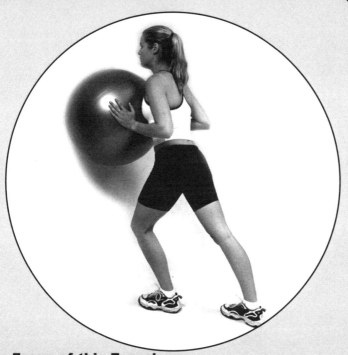

Main Focus of this Exercise:
• Increasing calf muscle flexibility.

How to perform this Exercise:
• Start in the same position as for a Wall Ball Calf Raise – 1 leg with the ball against the wall and you leaning your upper chest against it.
• Move your supporting leg far enough away from the wall so that you feel a stretch in your calf. Hold for 30 seconds and repeat on the other leg.

Notes:
• Be sure to keep your knee straight.

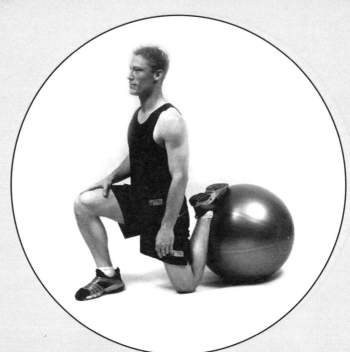

Main Focus of this Exercise:
• Increasing quadriceps and hip flexor muscle flexibility.
How to perform this Exercise:
• Place the top of one foot on top of the ball next to you so your toes are pointing behind you.
• Slowly move forward until the thigh of this leg is perpendicular with the floor.
• Lean your body back and bend slightly on your supportive knee until you feel a stretch down the front of the thigh on the ball.
• Hold for 30 seconds and repeat on your other thigh.
Notes:
• Be sure to keep your spine in a neutral alignment.

Lumbar Side Lying Stretch

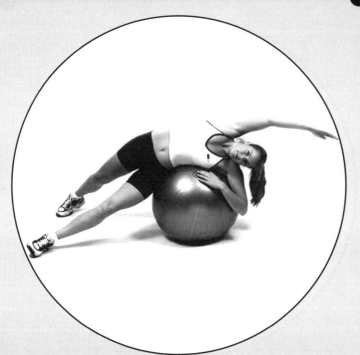

Main Focus of this Exercise:
• Increasing range of spinal lateral flexion.
• Increasing lateral spinal and lateral abdominal musculature flexibility.

How to perform this Exercise:
• Lie on your side with your arms outstretched over your head and the ball placed under the side of your lower abdomen.
• Separate your feet from each other to secure yourself on the ground.
• Allow your body to bend sideways within a comfortable range until you feel a stretch down the side of your body.
• Hold for 30 seconds and repeat on the other side of your body.

Notes:
• Only lean as far as comfortable without experiencing any pain.

Sitting Adductor/Hamstring Stretch

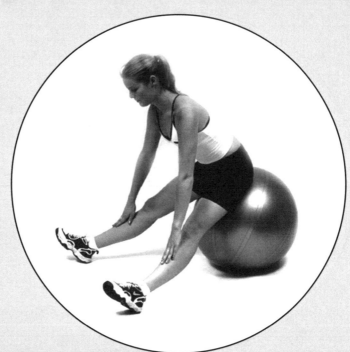

Main Focus of this Exercise:
• Increasing hamstring and adductor flexibility.
• Increasing lower spinal flexion mobility.

How to perform this Exercise:
• Sit on the ball with both legs stretched out straight with a wide stance.
• Lean forward slowly and reach for both ankles of your outstretched legs until your feel a stretch down the back and inside of each leg.
• Hold this for 30 seconds.

Notes:
• Only lean as far as comfortable without experiencing any pain.

Sitting Hamstring Stretch

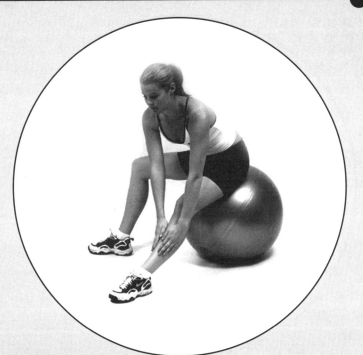

Main Focus of this Exercise:
• Increasing hamstring and gluteal flexibility.
• Increasing lower spinal flexion mobility.

How to perform this Exercise:
• Sit on the ball with one leg outstretched having a small bend in your knee.
• Keeping your back straight, lean forward and reach towards the ankle of the outstretched leg until you feel a stretch in the mid point of the back of your thigh.
• Hold this for 30 seconds and repeat on your other leg.

Notes:
• Only lean as far as comfortable without experiencing any pain.

Supine Hamstring Stretch

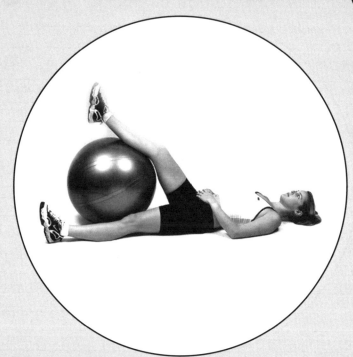

Main Focus of this Exercise:
• Increasing hamstring and gluteal flexibility.
How to perform this Exercise:
• Lie on your back with one leg outstretched on the ground and the other placed over a ball.
• Bring the ball closer to you until you feel a stretch in the mid point of the back of your thigh.
• Hold this for 30 seconds and repeat on your other leg.
Notes:
• Only lean as far as comfortable without experiencing any pain.

Sample Exercise Program - Level 1

Stage: Beginner
Focus: Whole Body -General base level strength and flexibility.
NB: To warm your body up, go for a walk around the block or if you have an exercise bike, cycle for 10 mins.

Exercise Name	Page	Sets	Repetitions
Warm Up	N/A	10 mins	
STRETCHES			
Supine Hamstring Stretch	86	1	30 seconds
Calf Stretch	81	1	30 seconds
Spinal Flexion Stretch	80	1	30 seconds
Hip Stretch	78	1	30 seconds
Lumbar Side Lying Stretch	83	1	30 seconds
EXERCISES			
Sitting on Ball	21	2	30 seconds
Ab Tucks	22	3	10 x each way
Trunk Rotations	29	2	10 x each way
Seated Circles	24	2	10 x each way
Seated One Leg Lifts	25	1	10 x each way
Prone Leg Abduction	31	2	10 x each way
Pelvic Lift with Support	32	1	10 x each way
Lying Side Rolls - Level 1	35	2	10 x each way
Wall Ball Squats - 2 Legs	39	2	10 x each way
Wall Ball Calf Raises - 2 Legs	40	2	10 x each way
REPEAT STRETCHES AS ABOVE		1	30 seconds

Remember: This is an example which may be suitable for a beginner with no previous injuries or medical conditions. Please consult a health professional before commencing this program.

Sample Exercise Program - Level 2

Stage: Intermediate
Focus: Whole Body
NB: To warm your body up, go for a walk around the block or if you have an exercise bike, cycle for 10 mins.

Exercise Name	Page	Sets	Repetitions
Warm Up	N/A	10 mins	
STRETCHES			
Hip Flexor Stretch	77	1	30 seconds
Seated Hamstring Stretch	85	1	30 seconds
Quadriceps Stretch	82	1	30 seconds
Lumbar Side Lying Stretch	83	1	30 seconds
Calf Stretch	81	1	30 seconds
EXERCISES			
Seated Circles	24	2	10 x each way
Seated Straight Leg Lifts - Level 1	27	3	10 x each way
Trunk Rotations - Level 2	30	2	10 x each way
Ab Squeeze	33		10 x each way
Seated Side Shifts - Level 2	34	2	10 x each way
Lying Side Rolls - Level 2	42	1	10 x each way
Supine Bridge	43	2	10 x each way
Prone Walk Forwards	44	1	10 x each way
Pelvic Lifts - Level 1	46	1	10 x each way
Wall Ball Calf Raises - 1 Leg	53	2	10 x each way
REPEAT STRETCHES AS ABOVE			

Remember: This program is not suitable for a beginner and assumes previous Swiss Ball experience. Please consult a health professional before commencing this program.

Sample Exercise Program - Level 3

Stage: Advanced
Focus: Whole Body
NB: To warm your body up, go for a walk around the block or if you have an exercise bike, cycle for 10 mins.

Exercise Name	Page	Sets	Repetitions
Warm Up	N/A	10 mins	
STRETCHES			
Ab Stretch	76	1	30 seconds
Hip Stretch	78	1	30 seconds
Quadriceps Stretch	82	1	30 seconds
Lumbar Side Lying Stretch	83	1	30 seconds
Sitting Adductor Hamstring Stretch	84	1	30 seconds
EXERCISES			
Seated Circles	24	2	10 x each way
Lying Side Rolls - Level 3	49	3	10 x each way
Reverse Curls with Ball	45	2	10 x each way
Supine Bridge with Dips	47		10 x each way
Side Lifts on Ball - Level 1	57	2	10 x each way
Push Ups Feet on Ball - Level 2	67	1	10 x each way
Pelvic Lifts with Tuck Ins - Level 3	70	2	10 x each way
Ball Dips Hands on Ball	60	1	10 x each way
Prone Back Extension - Level 2	51	2	10 x each way
Prone Tuck Ins	54	1	10 x each way
REPEAT STRETCHES AS ABOVE			

Remember: This program is not suitable for a beginner and assumes a significant amount of Swiss Ball experience. Please consult a health professional before commencing this program.

Personal Training Program

Day:_____

Date:_____

Workout Duration:_____

Start Time:_____

Body Parts Exercised:_____

_____

Today's Diet:
Poor ○ Moderate ○ Good ○ Excellent ○

Today's Mood:
Poor ○ Moderate ○ Good ○ Excellent ○

Energy Levels:
Poor ○ Moderate ○ Good ○ Excellent ○

Exercises Performed	Sets	Repetitions

Workout Intensity: _____%

Notes:_____

_____

_____

Personal Training Program

Day:_____

Date:_____

Workout Duration:_____

Start Time:_____

Body Parts Exercised:_____
_____

Today's Diet:
Poor ◯   Moderate ◯   Good ◯   Excellent ◯

Today's Mood:
Poor ◯   Moderate ◯   Good ◯   Excellent ◯

Energy Levels:
Poor ◯   Moderate ◯   Good ◯   Excellent ◯

Exercises Performed	Sets	Repetitions

Workout Intensity: _____%

Notes:_____
_____
_____

Personal Training Program

Day:_____

Date:_____

Workout Duration:_____

Start Time:_____

Body Parts Exercised:_____

_____

Today's Diet:
Poor ○ Moderate ○ Good ○ Excellent ○

Today's Mood:
Poor ○ Moderate ○ Good ○ Excellent ○

Energy Levels:
Poor ○ Moderate ○ Good ○ Excellent ○

Exercises Performed	Sets	Repetitions

Workout Intensity: _____%

Notes:_____

_____

_____

Personal Training Program

Day:_____
Date:_____

Workout Duration:_____
Start Time:_____

Body Parts Exercised:_____
_____

Today's Diet:
Poor ○   Moderate ○   Good ○   Excellent ○

Today's Mood:
Poor ○   Moderate ○   Good ○   Excellent ○

Energy Levels:
Poor ○   Moderate ○   Good ○   Excellent ○

Exercises Performed	Sets	Repetitions

Workout Intensity: _____%
Notes:_____
_____
_____

Personal Training Program

Day:_____
Date:_____

Workout Duration:_____
Start Time:_____

Body Parts Exercised:_____
_____

Today's Diet:
Poor ○ Moderate ○ Good ○ Excellent ○

Today's Mood:
Poor ○ Moderate ○ Good ○ Excellent ○

Energy Levels:
Poor ○ Moderate ○ Good ○ Excellent ○

Exercises Performed	Sets	Repetitions

Workout Intensity: _____%
Notes:_____
_____
_____

Personal Training Program

Day:_____
Date:_____

Workout Duration:_____
Start Time:_____

Body Parts Exercised:_____
_____

Today's Diet:
Poor ○ Moderate ○ Good ○ Excellent ○

Today's Mood:
Poor ○ Moderate ○ Good ○ Excellent ○

Energy Levels:
Poor ○ Moderate ○ Good ○ Excellent ○

Exercises Performed	Sets	Repetitions

Workout Intensity: _____%
Notes:_____
_____
_____

Personal Training Program

Day:_____

Date:_____

Workout Duration:_____

Start Time:_____

Body Parts Exercised:_____
_____

Today's Diet:

Poor ○ Moderate ○ Good ○ Excellent ○

Today's Mood:

Poor ○ Moderate ○ Good ○ Excellent ○

Energy Levels:

Poor ○ Moderate ○ Good ○ Excellent ○

Exercises Performed	Sets	Repetitions

Workout Intensity: _____%

Notes:_____
_____
_____